How Do I Know if I N

It can be frustrating to need help for emotio
problems and not understand what help is available or where to
find it. A big part of getting successful support to deal with a mental health problem is knowing what kind of help you need, what to expect, and how to speak up if you're not satisfied.

This guide is designed to help you get the services that are best for you. It covers some typical issues for which teens seek help. It also describes the kinds of people who provide help. And it describes the type of help they provide and the ways they provide it. After reading this guide you may have more questions. Talk with friends and with an adult you trust.

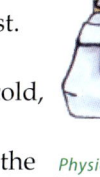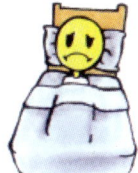

*Physical illness has physical symptoms.
Mental Illness has emotional symptoms.*

When people have a fever or a cold, they have a *physical* problem. Similarly, when people feel sad a lot of the time, can't concentrate in school, or feel overwhelmed by life's daily problems, they have what is called an *emotional* problem. Emotional problems can be mild—such as occasional sadness—or severe, such as weeks or months of feeling low.

Just as some physical illnesses or injuries can be helped through rest or physical therapy, emotional problems can be helped through self-help, counseling, and various kinds of therapy. Emotional problems, like physical problems, can also be treated with medication.

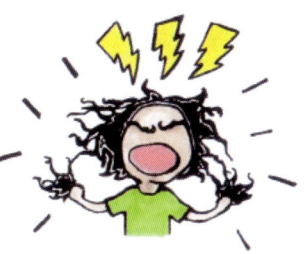

*Uncontrollable anger
is a mental health problem.*

Some kinds of medication can help balance your body chemistry to help you feel more in control of your feelings—somewhat like how other drugs can attack germs and help restore the balance needed for physical health.

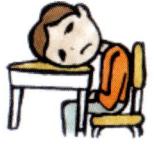

*Prolonged sadness
is a mental health problem.*

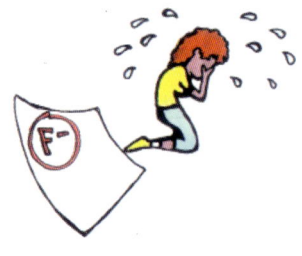

Temporary sadness over an event usually goes away.

So how do you know if you need to seek help?

We'll use depression as an example. That's the name people often use to describe everything from occasional sad moods to a serious disease requiring medical treatment. People who are depressed can feel sad, discouraged, angry, or hopeless. They may also feel irritable or exhausted, and lose interest and pleasure in daily activities.

Many people experience these feelings from time to time. However, if you have those kinds of feelings for weeks or months on end—and if they make it hard for you to get out of bed in the morning, socialize with friends, or enjoy yourself, or if everything seems to make you angry—you need to seek therapy. (More on therapy on pp. 6-9.)

A mental health professional can provide counseling that can help you feel better. If you're deeply depressed, and are not ready to tell an adult, tell a friend, and ask him or her to tell an adult.

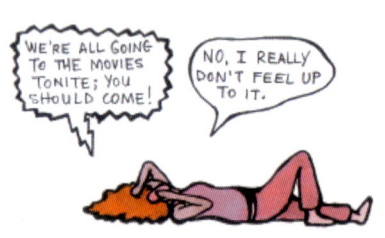

If you are too depressed to do regular activities, you may want to seek help.

But you don't have to be depressed, or feel like hurting yourself or someone else, to seek help. There are many other problems that can affect your ability to function and be happy, and for which you may need extra guidance and support. Perhaps you have conflicts with parents, siblings, or friends. Maybe someone in your family is suffering from mental or physical illness that is causing you stress. Maybe you can't concentrate enough in school to do as well as you know you can. You may have feelings of loneliness, anxiety, or isolation.

If something is interfering with your ability to feel productive or deal with the daily ups and downs of life, your best option is to connect with someone who can help.

What Kind of Help Is Best for Me?

There are many kinds of help out there. Below, we briefly describe some ways you can seek help for an emotional problem, from self-help to therapy to medication. We start with the most informal kinds of counseling you can get, and work up to the most formal or specialized.

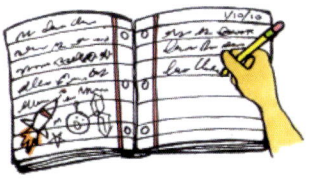

Writing can help you feel better.

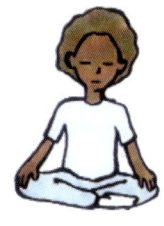

So can yoga...

Help yourself. First, there's **self-help**. Self-help means what it sounds like. You help yourself, often without any therapist at all. If you feel sad or angry because you're shy and can't make friends, you might read a book or magazine article on techniques for managing shyness. If the techniques work and you feel happier, you're doing great. There's probably no need to go to a counselor.

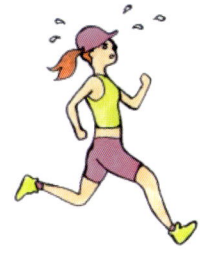

...or other physical activity, like running...

If you're upset, you can try writing down your feelings in a journal and describing the circumstances that are causing you to feel that way and what you can do about them. There's good evidence that writing about serious issues or trauma can help you release bottled-up feelings, see things differently, and improve your mental health. (See Anonymous's story on how writing can help, p. 18.)

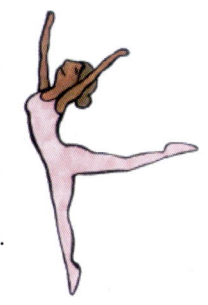

...or dance.

Get help from peers. The next level is getting help from friends. There are two main ways to do that: **informal help** from people you know, and something more formal called **peer self-help**.

Informal help from your friends means talking to friends about your problems. If you're feeling lonely, angry, or sad, confiding in a friend can help you feel better. You probably already know that, and already do it. Again, friends can help up to a certain point. But if you feel the problem is serious, you may need more help than your friends can give.

Self-help groups are a more formal way of getting help from people like you. Self-help groups are often run (or "facilitated") by an adult professional, but the real benefit comes from other teens in the group. So, for example, if you are cutting and want to stop, you might be able to find a self-help group of teens whose problems led them to cut themselves. They get together regularly to talk about problems in their lives and what strategies they use to try to stop cutting. (See Dina's story on peer support, p. 22.)

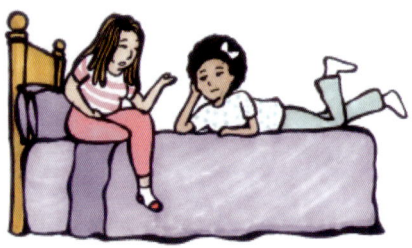
Feeling down? Talk with a friend.

Get help from a family member. It's sometimes hard for parents and teens to communicate because they seem to live in different worlds. And some parents just don't know how to be supportive. But even if you're wary of talking to family members, you probably have a good gut instinct about which parent or other family member, such as an aunt or uncle, could be helpful if you opened up to them. It may be scary to confide in them, but you may be surprised at how much they care, and may even learn that they struggled with similar issues at your age.

Get help from community members. There are lots of people in your day-to-day life who may be helpful to you. They may include school counselors, teachers, clergy, coaches, mentors, and any other adult who you trust and feel comfortable talking with about your problems.

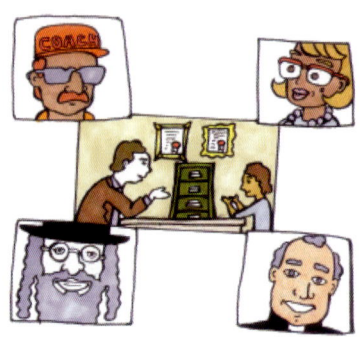
Mentors, teachers, clergy, and other caring adults can also be helpful.

Some of them, like a minister, may have training in counseling. Others, like a mentor, may not. But you're a good judge of how comfortable you are talking to them. If you start to feel better after talking with them, great. If not, they may be able to recommend someone else who could be helpful. Remember, it may take more than one talk session to help you feel better about yourself and your life, so give yourself and your counselor a chance.

Get help from professionals.
Therapists are professionals who are specially trained to help people with mental health issues. A therapist may be a psychiatrist, a psychologist, a social worker, or a psychiatric nurse. (See p. 17 for a more detailed description of these mental health professionals. And see p. 28 for Norman's story about therapy.)

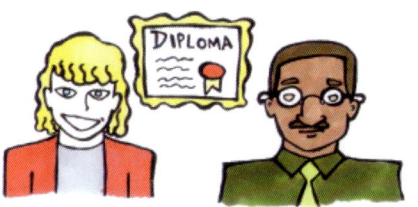
Many teens get help from talk therapy.

Whatever their training and background, most therapists do pretty much the same thing. They listen closely to how you describe what's making you feel bad or preventing you from achieving your goals. Then they work with you to help you change the thinking or feelings or actions that cause you problems or pain. (If you don't know how to find a mental health professional, but do have a regular medical doctor, talk to him or her. Doctors can offer advice and referrals, and also prescribe medication.)

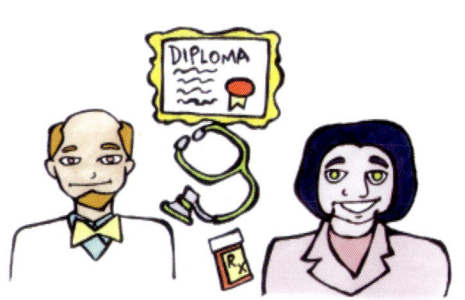
Medication is also helpful to many teens.

When They Say I Need Therapy or Counseling, What Do They Mean? What Kinds Are Available?

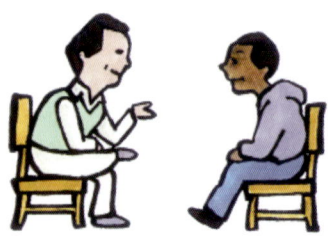

Counseling or therapy is a process where people explore their feelings, behavior, and what's going on in their lives. People go to counseling because they want to find ways to feel better and be more effective in their lives. (This kind of counseling is often called **therapy** or **psychotherapy**, or **psychological counseling** to show that it's different from something like job counseling.) If you get into formal counseling or therapy, you'll probably experience **individual therapy**, **group therapy**, or **family therapy**, or perhaps all of them. If your problems are severe, you may be **hospitalized**. We briefly describe these options below.

Individual Therapy: In individual therapy, you meet one-on-one with a counselor, usually at his or her office. You usually meet regularly, at least once a week, for anywhere from a few months to a year or longer, depending on the issues you're working on. You play an active role in defining the goals of your therapy with your counselor.

Group Therapy:
In group therapy, a group of people who are dealing with similar issues, such as depression or anxiety, meet 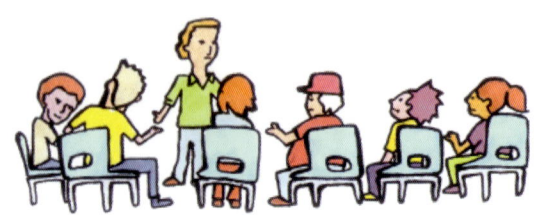 regularly with a therapist to talk about their struggles. In this way, teens can support and learn from each other as well as the therapist. Many people find that group therapy helps them to feel accepted and less isolated.

Peer self-help groups are one kind of group counseling, and they exist for many different issues. These groups may be self-directed, or led by a former participant who has recovered. In a formal setting like a drug treatment facility, groups are usually led by a mental health professional. Alcoholics and Narcotics Anonymous and Alateen (for teens who have family members with alcohol problems) are some of the most well-known self-help groups, but there are also groups for teen parents, teens with eating problems, teens who have lost a loved one, and many other issues.

Family Therapy: In family therapy, two or more members of a family will meet together and separately with a counselor to discuss conflicts, issues, and communication in the family. The counselor helps the family members deal with important issues without taking sides.

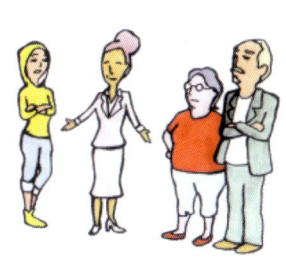

Hospitalization: If you have severe emotional or mental health problems, such as strong feelings of hopelessness or that you may hurt yourself or someone else, or that you're losing control, or that you cannot quit drugs without more structure and support, you may want to be hospitalized or referred to a drug rehab center.

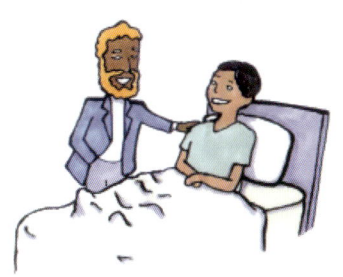

Hospitalization (which is also called "in-patient" treatment because you stay *in* the hospital) gives you a chance to get intensive services. For example, you may participate in individual, group, family, or peer counseling every day, as well as be given medication, to see what helps you most.

Once you leave the hospital, or instead of staying there, you may be referred to **outpatient** or **day treatment** services. That means you'll get similar intensive services, usually at a hospital or treatment center, but without having to stay there overnight. (See Dina's story on attending a day treatment center for depression, p. 22.)

What If I Feel Uncomfortable in Therapy?

One goal of therapy is to help you solve some problems, and to think differently about the problems you can't solve, so you can manage them better and don't blame yourself for them. When that happens, your self-esteem usually starts to rise.

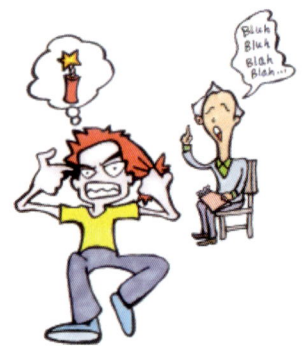
Sometimes therapy is hard.

However, at first it can be very uncomfortable to look at problems in your life and talk about them in peer groups or with adult professionals. Boys, in particular, often get the message that it's not "manly" to ask for help. Of course, it is admirable to take responsibility for yourself. But part of taking responsibility for yourself is acknowledging your feelings, and getting help when that is what you need to feel better.

Before your first visit to a therapist you might feel worried about what might happen at the session. You may feel anxious that the therapist will think your problem is strange. You may think you don't really need help because your issue isn't that big. These feelings are common. But remember that therapists are used to dealing with all sorts of issues. If an issue is worrying you, that makes it important to a therapist.

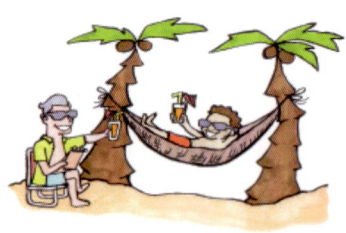
And sometimes it feels great.

It is important in therapy to gradually face hard issues about yourself or others in your life. That can be very difficult. Sometimes the best therapist is the one who is demanding and occasionally makes you feel pretty uncomfortable. The times that you want "out" of therapy or feel you need another therapist may be when you're making the most progress. At those times, it can be hard to figure out whether you don't like the *therapist,* or whether you don't like the *issues* he or she is asking you to think about. You need to be able to trust that your therapist has your best interests at heart, even if he or she sometimes makes you feel uncomfortable.

Can I Change Therapists?

If you begin to feel uncomfortable in therapy, or feel that you are not making progress, don't just jump to another therapist. Discuss these issues with your therapist. A good therapist should be willing to talk with you about treatment issues, and about whether the therapy is meeting your needs. A good therapist should also be willing to consider changing the way he or she works with you.

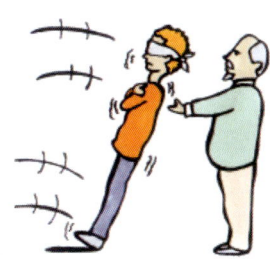

Trust is important in therapy.

It takes time to develop trust in a new relationship and to comfortably share feelings, so give your therapist and yourself some time. But if you've given it an honest shot and still don't feel you can trust your therapist, or if you don't feel like you're making progress over time, you may need a change.

It can be helpful, before starting therapy, to check out more than one therapist. If it's possible for you to do so, meet with two or three therapists, ask them how they work, and try to get a sense of how comfortable you feel with each. (See Norman's story on p. 28 about changing therapists.)

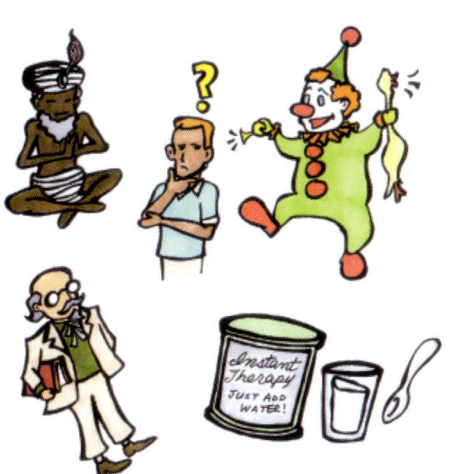

It can be hard to find a good therapist.

Even if you are assigned a therapist, you can ask to be changed to a new one if, after working together for a time, you feel that person is not right for you.

9

Privacy

When you talk with someone about your private issues, you probably don't want them sharing that information without your permission. Ask the therapist in your first session what sort of confidentiality he or she can provide. For example, will the therapist share your conversations with your parents? With other people in the agency? Will the therapist share some kinds of information, but not others?

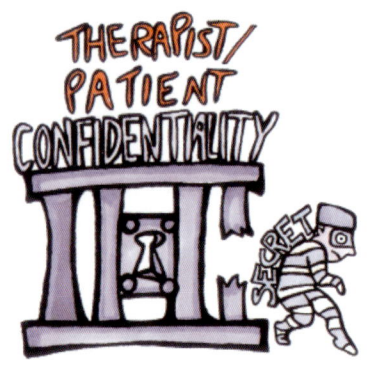

Talk with your therapist about what is confidential and what is not.

In general, people who offer licensed psychological counseling (psychiatrists, psychologists, and social workers) can offer much more confidentiality than informal counselors, like teachers and mentors (who may not be legally required to keep your conversations confidential). You need to ask them who they share information with and why—and then make your own decisions about what you want to reveal.

Note that even if everything else you say is confidential, therapists are required to tell others if you threaten to harm yourself or others.

A Few Words About "Cognitive-Behavioral" Therapy

In addition to the forms of therapy described here (individual counseling, family counseling, etc.) there are many *kinds* of therapy. One kind that has been shown to work well with teens for some issues is cognitive-behavioral therapy. That's a fancy name for a pretty simple technique.

"Cognitive" means "thinking." In the first part of cognitive-behavioral therapy you work to replace self-defeating or self-destructive thoughts with more helpful thoughts. For example, if you're failing in school, you may think, "I'm sure to fail every class." But if you can change your *thinking* to, "I failed because I didn't study," and, "If I study for my next test, I may do better," then you're half way to a good change.

But just changing your thinking isn't enough. You also have to change what you *do*. In the example about failing classes, if you change your *behavior* too (that is, you actually do some studying)—then things will start to change for the better.

Therapists use cognitive-behavioral methods to help you change negative thinking and actions into more positive approaches.

When Can Medication Be Helpful?

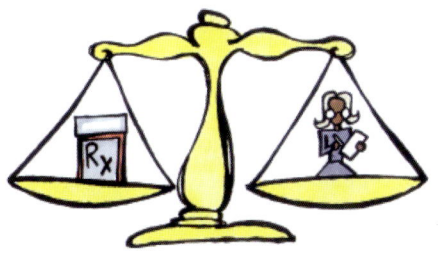

Effective therapy often requires the right balance of talk and medication.

Just as doctors prescribe medication to treat physical illness, doctors also sometimes prescribe medication to treat emotional problems, such as depression.

There is medication for all kinds of emotional problems, but the most common issues for which teens get medication include depression, having trouble focusing (ADD, ADHD), and severe acting out or uncontrolled behavior (ODD).

One medication may work for some people but not for others. For example, many people use anti-depressants and feel the medication changed their lives by lifting their depression. But there are others for whom the medication has not worked as well.

That's why you need to ask questions and discuss your concerns with your therapist when you start any therapy program, especially one that involves medication. Medication may be necessary and effective, but you and your therapist need to give careful thought to whether you need it and, if you do, to how it can be combined with

11

talk therapy and other support.

Medication can take several weeks to start working in your system, and how well it will work and what side effects you feel cannot be precisely predicted. Over time you, your therapist (and the doctor who prescribed the medication) will evaluate the effectiveness of the drug and make changes until you figure out what works best. Your input will be very important because you are the only one who really knows how it is affecting you.

It is important to take medication exactly as prescribed, and then to notice how it makes you feel. If it doesn't seem to be working or has unpleasant side effects (or makes you feel suicidal, which can happen in rare cases), you may need to be put on another medication or get a smaller or larger dose, or go off medication altogether. But since getting the right medication and the right dose to reduce your symptoms is complicated, it is very important that you work closely with your therapist and psychiatrist.

When you are feeling better you may feel tempted to reduce the dose or stop taking medication altogether. But making those changes by yourself can make you feel sick. Don't stop or change the amount of medication you take without first talking to your doctor about the safest way to do it. And, just as it's important to monitor your reactions when you start medication, you want to monitor your reactions to reducing or going off of medication to make sure you're getting a result that's helpful to you.

The bottom line: You need to play an active role in developing a treatment plan that works for you, and in monitoring how the medication and other supports are affecting you.

Remember, some problems can be treated by self-help and informal counseling with adults you trust. But for other problems you may need help from therapists and sometimes from medication, or even hospitalization. Don't be afraid to seek help if you feel you need it. Don't "tough it out." The best reason to seek help early is that it may prevent problems from becoming more severe, and will help you get better sooner, which you and everyone who cares about you will be grateful for.

Mental Health Terms You May Want to Know

You may have heard many of these terms and be unsure of what they mean. This list is designed to make you more familiar with common mental health terms and to explain what they mean.

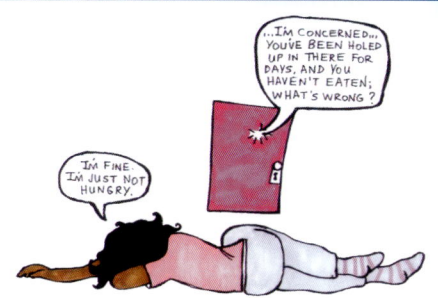
Professional help can ease depression and make you feel better.

Depression is the name people use to describe everything from occasional sad moods to a serious disease requiring medical treatment. Depression can be caused by chemical imbalances in your brain, or by traumatic events in your life, such as abuse, the loss of someone dear to you, or conflict with parents, teachers, or friends. People who are depressed can feel sad, discouraged, hopeless, or angry. They can feel irritable, lose interest and pleasure in daily activities, and feel worthless and alone. If you have those kinds of feelings for weeks or months on end, you need to seek professional therapy.

Since the cause of depression can be complicated, it's often important to have more than one form of treatment. For example, talking with a therapist can help you deal with the effects of problems in your life, resolve conflict issues, and learn coping skills. And medication may help with chemical imbalances in the brain.

Even mild depression can lead to thoughts of suicide and suicide attempts. Many people have occasional thoughts of suicide when they are very upset, such as after breaking up with a boyfriend or girlfriend. But if you are feeling depressed and continue to think about hurting yourself and planning ways to end your life, tell someone and get professional help. If you won't tell an adult, tell a friend.

ADD (or ADHD) is another common mental health problem among children and teens.

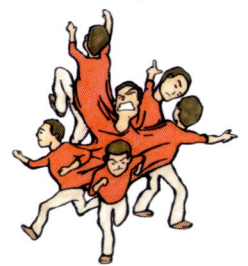
Medication may reduce ADHD symptoms.

Like depression, it's complicated. But the letters provide a pretty good clue: they stand for **A**ttention **D**eficit

13

MENTAL HEALTH TERMS

(**H**yperactivity) **D**isorder. People with ADHD have a very hard time (much harder than most) focusing on a single task or paying attention or staying still long enough to get something done. This problem is also often treated with medications.

ODD stands for **O**ppositional **D**efiant **D**isorder. It means that you are often defiant or hostile toward adults and sometimes your peers, and you often feel very angry and frustrated over things that don't seem to bother other people all that much.

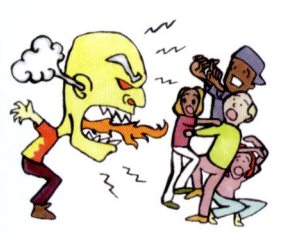
Talk therapy may help you control anger.

Of course, you may have good reasons to be angry. But if your anger is preventing you from being happy or working toward your goals (for example, because you're often getting disciplined at school, or taking illegal drugs to calm down), then you have a problem that you need to work on. ODD is typically treated in talk therapy and/or with medication.

Anxiety problems: Everyone gets anxious from time to time and a bit of anxiety can help you stay alert and perform better. But if you're feeling nervous and anxious a lot of the time, and it makes it hard to do your schoolwork or do stuff with friends, then you may have an anxiety disorder. There are different kinds of anxiety disorders. For example:

Social anxiety means you get really scared in social situations. It's so bad that you avoid social situations.

Post-traumatic stress disorder (PTSD) is an anxiety disorder that comes from a very traumatic event like a serious accident or a sexual assault. You may have "flashbacks," upsetting memories, and trouble sleeping.

Obsessive Compulsive Disorder (OCD) is an anxiety disorder in which you have lots of unwanted thoughts (obsessions) and the urge to do things, like counting or washing your hands, over and over again (compulsions). Doing things over and over again may temporarily control the bad thoughts or feelings, but it won't make them go away. Medication, therapy, and self-help groups can be helpful in treating OCD.

A *panic attack* is something that happens suddenly, without warning, and lasts a few minutes. During a panic attack you feel intense fear and extreme anxiety. You also

MENTAL HEALTH TERMS

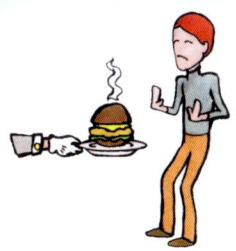

Anorexia and bulimia can be life threatening. Get help!

have physical sensations like heart pounding, dry mouth, feeling short of breath and like you're losing control.

Anorexia and bulimia are
eating disorders. People who have **anorexia** become obsessed with getting rid of any fat on their body, and they eat less and less (and sometimes also exercise more and more). If they keep it up too long, they can actually starve to death. **Bulimia** is purposely throwing up your food before digesting it. Regularly throwing up food can cause its own health problems over time, like rotting teeth. And if the problem is related to anorexia, it can also contribute to starvation. Anorexia and bulimia are serious problems that require professional help and support.

Self-esteem means how you
feel about yourself. In general, low self-esteem means you feel bad about yourself. You may tell yourself you are bad or not worthy of attention or love or having good things happen to you. Very low self-esteem often leads to depression, cutting, or substance abuse. Having a problem like that can push your self-esteem even lower.

Healthy self-esteem means you basically feel positive about who you are. However, good self-esteem is not just having a high opinion of yourself. Being arrogant, boastful, bullying others, or feeling entitled to more than other people is not healthy self-esteem.

Self-mutilation is when a
person harms herself to create feelings of pain. A common form of self-mutilation is **cutting**, where a person cuts herself (or himself) to cause pain and bleeding. People who self-mutilate sometimes get pleasure or emotional release from physical pain,

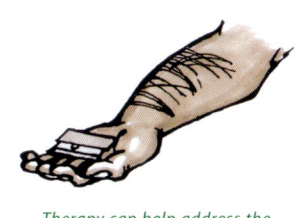

Therapy can help address the issues that lead to cutting.

similar to what some people get from using drugs. Self-mutilation can cause physical problems such as scarring and infection. But, more importantly, it's a sign that something else is not right in your life. Therapy and even self-help groups can help you identify what's bothering you and begin to deal with the real problem.

Substance abuse means
using drugs in ways that are harmful to you. You can abuse legal drugs (like caffeine, alcohol, cigarettes, and prescription medication, like Ritalin). Or

15

MENTAL HEALTH TERMS

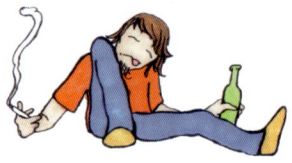

Self-medication can have unpleasant side effects.

you can abuse illegal drugs, like marijuana or cocaine. Substance abuse can be especially hard to deal with because some substances are addictive or strongly habit-forming, which makes quitting them very difficult. Regular use of some drugs can actually change your brain chemistry, so that it is harder for your brain to make the chemicals that naturally make you feel happy. Plus, using drugs usually makes it more difficult to think rationally, so it becomes harder to know that you have a problem.

Child abuse can cause many of the mental health problems described above. Child abuse includes things adults do to kids, like harsh physical punishments (that's **physical abuse**). It also includes inappropriate sexual contact, like touching the private parts of a child or youth, or forcing the child to touch them (that's **sexual abuse**). It also includes

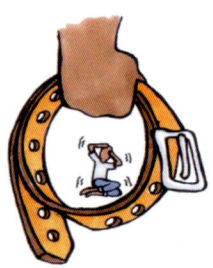

Harsh punishments are physical abuse.

treating the child very badly, such as constantly telling them they are worthless, or letting them watch one parent hit or abuse the other (that's **emotional abuse**).

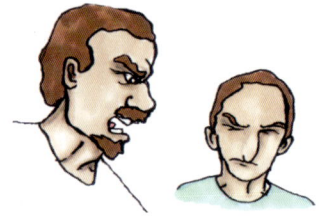

Constant criticism can be emotional abuse.

Abuse can also include what adults *don't* do. For example, if a parent fails to provide food, or leaves young children alone for long periods, that's **neglect**. Children have a right not to be abused or neglected. If you have been abused or neglected, you probably need help to deal with the feelings and the behavior that have resulted from it.

If you or your brothers or sisters are being abused or neglected *now*, your

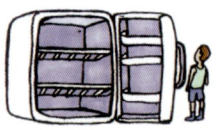

Failure to provide essentials like food is neglect.

whole family may need help. Many agencies can provide services to help parents find better, more loving ways to raise children. In extreme cases, children may be removed from the family and put into foster care to protect them until their parents get their act together.

16

The People Who Help

The four main types of licensed mental health professional that you may work with are psychologists, social workers, psychiatrists, and psychiatric nurse practitioners. Here's a brief description of those jobs.

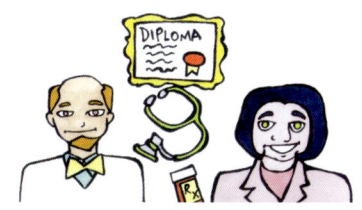

Psychologists and **social workers** are trained mainly to do psychological counseling or therapy. That means they help with problems of feelings, relationships, habits, and behaviors. There are many different kinds of psychologists and social workers.

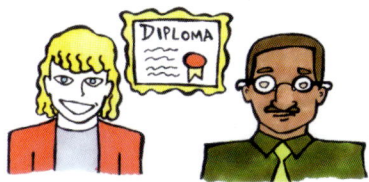

Some psychologists and social workers have extra training in very specialized areas, such as substance abuse, or teen issues, or working with whole families. If you have a specific problem, it may help to go to someone who has training or experience in those types of issues.

Psychiatrists are medical doctors with special training in mental health issues. In theory, that means they can help you with "talk therapy," just like psychologists and social workers. Psychiatrists are the ones who will prescribe medication when it is needed.

If you are referred to a mental health center, you will probably be assigned to a therapist who is not a psychiatrist for talk therapy. If you and your therapist decide that you should consider medication, the psychiatrist's role will be to evaluate you by discussing your situation with you and your therapist, and prescribing the appropriate medication.

The psychiatrist will continue to see you from time to time to evaluate your progress on the medication. He or she will depend on you to report how the medication makes you feel so he or she can decide whether to continue with the same medication, change it, decrease or increase it, or discontinue it.

Psychiatric nurse practitioners can evaluate your emotional problems, offer therapy, and also prescribe medication, under the supervision of a psychiatrist.

17

Self-Help—True Story by a Teen

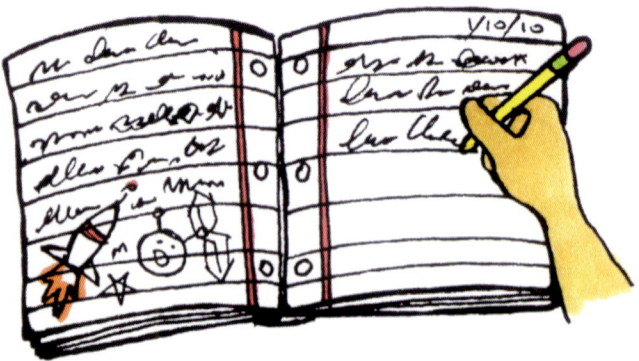

My Journal Saved My Life

By Anonymous

When I was in the 9th grade, my mom lost her job and we could no longer afford our apartment. My dad had left us and wasn't giving us financial support. I was really depressed because I was concerned about my next meal and where I would sleep (and you can imagine how my mom felt).

I wasn't really talking to anyone about what I was going through, which wasn't a good feeling. But I eventually started keeping a journal and that really helped me out. I gained a better understanding of myself and how to handle emotional problems through writing in my diary and re-reading it.

Writing allows my emotions to pour out of my emotional storage bag, my heart. Once it's opened and my feelings are released, I am at ease. But when I'm going through a hard situation and my emotional storage bag is closed, I feel a lot of pressure. I worry that I may eventually explode or take out my pain on someone else if the pressure is not released.

At one point, my father was the main source of that pressure. He made everything a nightmare for me. He was physically abusive to my mother when they lived together. I hated him for hurting her. Sometimes I wished he would die. But those were just angry thoughts. I didn't really mean it. I always thought that I should try to forgive him because he was my father and it was the "Christ-like" thing to do.

I felt like I was basically on "No-Man's Island." I had just started high school and was getting to know people there. I couldn't talk with my friends about what was going on at home. I didn't feel like I could trust anyone. I felt pushed into isolation.

Toward the end of the school year, my father stopped helping my mom with the rent. She couldn't afford the apartment alone, so we moved to a two-room basement apartment a few blocks away. It was small and I didn't like it, but it was the only thing we could afford.

Apart from getting good grades, nothing in my life was good. I felt suicidal. Life to me was not worth living because everything was so complicated. At 14, I just couldn't understand why I had to deal with so much.

I made it through 9th grade, but I felt terrible. My father was still calling my mother even though they weren't living together. On one particular summer night, he called and they got into a heated conversation. He threatened to kill her. I think my mother was worried, but she didn't show it. I felt horrible. The thought of losing my mother terrified me. After I heard what happened, I wrote in my diary for the very first time. It was really just a plain notebook, but I felt like I had to write in it. I had to release what I was feeling.

When I began to write in my journal, I was finally able to detail what was happening with my parents. Although my diary couldn't offer advice, it was such a relief to get my emotions down on paper.

Although my diary couldn't offer advice, it was such a relief to get my emotions down on paper.

I began to write in my journal almost every day. After I poured out everything in those entries I felt much better, though I still worried about what would happen to my mother. I would open up completely in my diary. It's almost like my head went from heavy to empty, especially when I wrote about my father's behavior. When I wrote my angry thoughts, my mind was less stressed. It's like I told someone my feelings and they offered to listen. I didn't feel sad or suicidal anymore.

Eventually I realized that writing was helping me cope with my father. In fact, I think my diary saved me. Whenever something bad happened, I would write about it. Before I had my diary, I would just sit and cry and hope for the best. Sometimes I prayed, too. But writing helped me the most. A few days after making an entry, I would go back to read what I wrote. Re-reading the journal entries still made me angry as I remembered those awful situations, but the feelings of hate toward my father had left me.

Thankfully, my home life eventually got better. My mother got a job and we started getting back on our feet. Mommy said that as soon as she got enough money, we would move to a better apartment. My dad is now incarcerated because of other offenses, and I don't fear him hurting my mom anymore. We correspond with him by mail.

My journal helped me to let go, and as a result, I've changed a lot. I understand myself better now. I've also been able to write about things besides my difficult home life. When I re-read my diary a few times, I noticed that I write about sports a lot. That led me to join a couple of sports teams in high school.

I've also written a lot about boys. I kept a record of the guys I dated and how I felt about them. Reading these entries now, I realize that for a long time I was looking for a father figure, not a boyfriend. I noticed how the guys I would go for were usually older and more

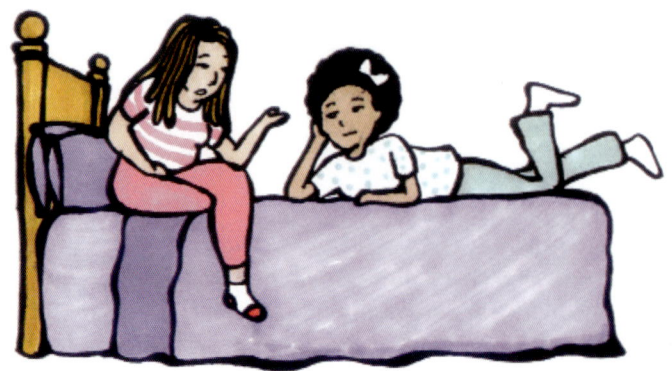

serious. I felt like I always wanted a guy who could give me fatherly advice as well as intimacy, probably because I lacked a father who was consistent in my life. But I see things a lot differently now.

Re-reading my journal entries, I realize that I'm a capable person and I don't need a boyfriend who would be like a second father. For instance, in one of my entries, I wrote about Ron. He was definitely a "father-figure," but I realized I never liked how I felt around him. I didn't feel I could fully voice my opinion around him because he had a serious, gruff tone that scared me. Scanning my entries on Ron, I began to figure out that I might be better off dating a guy who could be a boyfriend and a friend at the same time, a person who isn't always serious. My journal helped me figure out that I wanted someone to have fun with.

When I wrote my angry thoughts, my mind was less stressed.

My journal was my best friend. It made me think and helped me come up with different ways to handle problems by myself. I still write in it, but I feel more comfortable now talking about my problems with a few chosen friends. My diary has made that a lot easier as well. By writing down how I feel about something before talking about it, I'm a lot more clear about what I want to say. I don't have to hustle to figure out my feelings right before I speak.

I now have more than three years of my life recorded in a book. I'm so glad to have my journal. I recently named it "Precious," because that's how I feel about all the thoughts it contains.

The writer was in high school when she wrote this story. She later attended Lehman College.

Group Therapy and Peer Support—True Story by a Teen

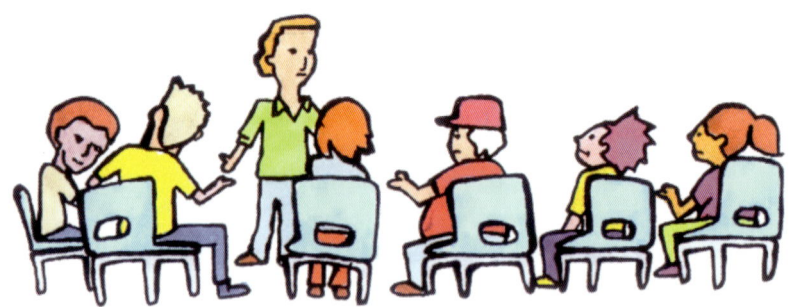

How My Group Helped Me Fight Depression

By Dina Spanbock

"Last night I was a four and now I'm a two," one kid said. I didn't know what he was talking about. As Steve, the program coordinator, called on other teens in the group, a dozen of them said similar things, adding on a goal for the day at the end. Then Steve turned to me. "All right, Dina—now I'm going to ask you to introduce yourself, and tell us a little about why you're here," he said.

Now? Just like that? What was I supposed to say? That I was here because my dad died and I had stopped going to school and I needed to do something? And I had to say it to a room full of strangers?

I had struggled with depression and anxiety on and off for nearly five years. I only talked to a few of my close friends about it, but by sophomore year of high school, everyone at school could tell something was going on. Ever since my dad had died in the middle of freshman year, I'd been missing school a lot, sometimes for weeks at a time.

But if anyone asked where I'd been, I just said I hadn't been feeling well. After a while, they learned to stop asking. I avoided the subject at all costs. Sometimes, that was why I didn't go to school. I was ashamed and didn't want to have to explain to anyone that I was depressed. I was sure they would've been puzzled by the idea that living was so incredibly difficult.

But living was difficult for me. Depression makes everything difficult. It takes over your body, mind, and spirit. Simple things like getting up in the morning can take so much effort that by the time you do it, you're so tired that you need to lie back down.

By the middle of my junior year, I was sick of struggling every day, always having trouble getting to school. I decided something had to change. With the help of my psychiatrist, I decided to go to Four Winds, a psychiatric treatment center in Westchester, New York, that has programs specifically for adolescents. I wanted to be rid of my depression, or at least learn how to deal with it. I ended up learning a lot more than I expected.

I started commuting to Four Winds each day to take part in a three-month program. When I got there on the first day, I waited anxiously for my group therapy to begin. This was the morning check-in group, the staff told me, during which we were supposed to say how our night was and choose a goal for the day, anything from talking more in groups to not arguing with staff.

Depression makes everything difficult. It takes over your body, mind, and spirit.

When they asked me to introduce myself, I spoke softly. "Um, I'm Dina. I'm here because I guess I've just been having, um, a lot of trouble, like, getting to school lately…"

Some of the other teens asked questions. I liked the easy ones.

"Where are you from?"

"Manhattan."

Then someone asked why I wasn't going to school.

"Well, my, uh, father died a couple years ago, and since then I, it's been, um, kind of hard for me to, um, go to school because of… depression," I said.

Steve explained that the numbers corresponded to feelings, one being great, five being in crisis. He asked me what I was at the moment. "Um, about a…a three?" I said, meaning that I was so-so.

They moved on to the next person, and I became a bit closer to a 2.5.

We spent most of our time at Four Winds in various groups. Each group had a different aim, like discussing family conflict or medications. In the psychodrama group, we acted out situations and figured out how to respond. There was even a sharing group, where we had the opportunity to show other participants anything that we did or made, like art or photography. There was school for a couple of hours a day. And after lunch, we usually had a bit of downtime where we just hung around and talked.

As the days went by and the routines and people became more familiar, I became more comfortable there. I talked more about my feelings in group therapy. I began to give advice as well as take it. During sharing group, I sang. But I had to push myself to do all this. I still felt ashamed of being depressed and being at a treatment center.

One day, after a few weeks in the program, I woke up and my mood was pretty low. On the train to Four Winds, I only felt worse. By the time group therapy began, I was feeling suicidal. I surprised myself by telling everyone at group that morning. I had sometimes told people about being suicidal once I felt better, but I had never told anyone I was suicidal while I still felt it. I was nervous that people would get really worried about me and just feel bad.

I was feeling suicidal. I surprised myself by telling everyone at group that morning.

Other kids in the group started saying things like, "You're such a great person," and, "We would be so upset if you died," and, "Think about your family and friends." It was nice to hear I was wanted, but it didn't help much. I still felt terrible, and their words did not make me want to live.

Then a girl named Melanie spoke. "But when you're suicidal, you're selfish. You're not thinking about all the other people. You're so upset that nothing else matters. You can't worry about how other people would feel. You're too focused on how you're feeling."

I was in shock. All I could say was, "Yeah, exactly!" She knew what I was feeling even better than I did. She knew it and she could say it. I'd never really put what I felt into words before, but whatever I was feeling, I didn't think it was OK to feel that way.

Melanie helped me realize what I was feeling: selfish. But not the kind of selfish you can help feeling, not the kind of selfish I should blame myself for feeling. Being suicidal meant all you could think about was how awful you felt, not about how it affected anyone else.

Melanie's words made me realize that it was OK to feel that way at times. Sure, it wasn't ideal to feel so down and I should work to change it if I could, but I realized I also shouldn't beat myself up inside for being depressed. It was just the way I felt. I couldn't help it; I didn't ask for it.

Her words also made me feel a connection. Not just with Melanie, but with everyone who had been through depression. I realized that we all shared something special that no one else could understand. It was almost like I was part of a worldwide club filled with strangers who I would instantly feel comfortable talking to.

I could talk about my trouble getting to school, or being suicidal, or all the times I had hidden anxiety attacks in school. Talking to members of this "club" at Four Winds, hearing their experiences and relating mine to theirs, allowed me to be happy for the first time in years. It helped me to get things off my chest, and my new friends' understanding responses helped even more. I had a support system. The feeling of complete loneliness withered away.

After that, when new people came to the program, I tried to make them comfortable. I showed them around, reassured them that this was a good place, asked them about their problems and often responded with my own story. I think it helped them, knowing they weren't alone.

We had fun, too. You might not expect it in a place filled with depressed people, but we could laugh and smile and have a good time. My friends Rob and Zoe and I used to go down to school every morning and afternoon together. But we didn't walk down the road from the main building to the school. We shuffled.

We shuffled our feet slowly but surely, all the while reminding each other and ourselves, "Shuffle!" It started out as a way to stall, but it became a way to make fun of ourselves. We joked about being mental patients, shuffling along the road rather than walking like "normal" people. Once a van drove by as we were shuffling along. "Ha ha, that van driver must know he's in a mental hospital now," Zoe laughed.

"Shuffle!" Rob shouted.

In unison, Zoe and I replied, "Shuffle!" And we continued, shuffling along to school.

In a way, our shuffling was the perfect metaphor for my entire experience at Four Winds. I took small steps, one at a time, and in the end, with others' help and support, I got to my destination. I learned to accept my depression.

I also learned ways to cope with my depression, like opening up and talking to people about my issues while they were going on, not just afterward. I learned breathing exercises to help with my anxiety. And I learned that in order to feel less depressed, I needed to stop isolating myself and get involved in activities even when I didn't feel like it.

I had a support system. The feeling of complete loneliness withered away.

Most of all, I was learning to feel comfortable in my own skin, comfortable with the fact that I was struggling, and even able to laugh and make fun of it. We all embraced our issues as a part of ourselves. In a way, I even began to be happy that I had struggled so hard, because it allowed me to go to Four Winds and meet these wonderful people I connected with so intensely. It was a connection that could only be made by fully understanding and talking about our hard times.

Leaving Four Winds after three months was extremely difficult. I loved my friends there. I didn't want to leave that world, where people understood and accepted my many issues, and where everyone could relate to me. But my program was finished and it was time to go.

One day soon after I left, I was sitting in the student lounge back at my old school, talking with some classmates. Somehow we had gotten onto the subject of medications people were on, I think because someone mentioned his attention deficit disorder.

"Ah, medication. So helpful," said Josh.

"I've been on everything," I said. "All my craziness will get you to at least try just about everything. I never used to think of depression as a mental illness, but that's what it is. I mean, clearly, with all these meds, I'm mentally ill," I said, smiling. I was so used to it being normal to talk like this among my Four Winds friends that I had forgotten other people don't see it this way.

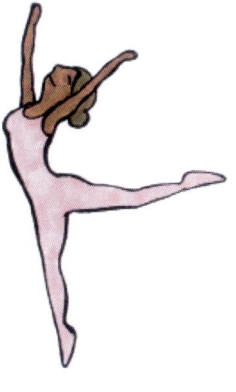

No one said anything and an awkward silence filled the room. "And there goes my anxiety, skyrocketing," I thought as I sat uncomfortably in the silence. But although it was awkward and I felt anxious, I'm glad I spoke about it. Hopefully, next time someone talks about mental illness with my classmates, particularly depression, they won't feel quite as uncomfortable.

Depression isn't a subject people talk about openly very often. When they do, it's usually very serious. But that's not how I talk about it now. I'm no longer ashamed of my struggles and I don't want to go back to feeling that way. If it comes up, I tell my story, no matter who's there. I let people know that there's nothing to hide or be ashamed of. I do this in the hope that some day, depression will become less taboo.

I know depression doesn't just go away. It continues to be a struggle for me and probably will be for quite some time. Luckily, I have the support of my friends from Four Winds who I've stayed in touch with. And although I'm still learning how to cope with my depression, I've taken the most important step—I've accepted that it's a part of me.

Dina was 19 when she wrote this story.
She later went to college in Massachusetts.

Individual Therapy—True Story by a Teen

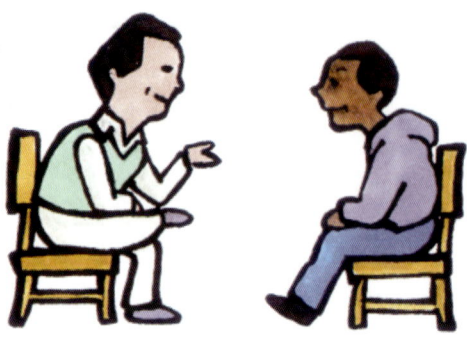

Don't Keep It Inside: Talk It Out

By Norman B.

In the past four years, I've had four different therapists. Each time I went to one I was hoping to find someone who cared enough to tell me the things I did wrong and help me go about changing them. But until I found my fourth therapist, I was lost inside my own world.

I went to my first therapist at age 12. At the time, my life was filled with chaos, and I didn't know who to talk to or how to handle it. My dad was in jail, my mother and I weren't talking, and in a little more than a year several family members had died. All the feelings I had began to build up inside, and I felt like I was drowning in my emotions.

Sometimes I would cry like a baby over all the death in my family. Other times I'd feel angry and confused. I didn't trust anyone, especially my family, and I thought people were saying negative things about me. I started to disrespect my elders, steal, stay out late, and fail in school.

Things got so bad that I was sent to two different group homes. At the homes I pretended to feel better about myself, but being there made me feel like more of a failure and like I didn't deserve to live. I really needed someone to talk to. I needed someone to show me that there was still hope for me and to help me realize that everything that was going on wasn't all my fault.

I went to one therapist after another. But my therapists didn't ask how I was really feeling, which was what I wanted. Instead they just skimmed the surface of the problems and offered me useless advice like, "Watch your temper," or "Try to fit in."

But my fourth therapist, Dr. Kaputer, was different. She didn't talk to me like I was a toddler. And she hardly ever talked about herself. She didn't act like I had to take her advice just because she went to school for it. And if I ever forgot to come for an appointment, she'd call to remind me. That alone made me feel like she really cared. Slowly I began to open up and tell her more about myself.

I remember one time I was hit in the face by another resident of my group home, and it left a mark under my eye. From that day until the mark went away, I was picked on. It was like I was garbage in a dumpster, and the residents were the seagulls—just picking and picking at me until there was practically nothing there. I pretended that what they said didn't hurt, but it did. They would say things like, "Norm's a punk," or, "Check out big Norm with the black eye." Even though it was a joke to them, it wasn't to me.

> **I needed someone to show me that there was still hope for me and to help me realize that everything wasn't all my fault.**

At first I didn't want to talk to Dr. K about the fight. I didn't care how it started, or the consequences I had to suffer. It was the reactions I got from people that bothered me, and that was what I wanted to talk about. She asked me how I felt about all the attention I was getting. Of course I said I was angry and didn't like it. But then she repeated the question, explaining that she wanted to know how I *really* felt about people making fun of me.

Again I tried to work my way around the question, but I didn't get far because she asked again. Finally, I told her, "It hurts so bad until I can't describe it," which is what she wanted to hear—and what I needed to say. How I really felt. After that session, it became easier for me to express my true feelings.

Another time someone spread a rumor saying that I had sex with one of the residents. That whole thing went around the entire campus infecting people's brains like crack. And it lasted for weeks. Some of the residents would say, "Your roommate said you had sex with another resident," or, "Yo, I heard you was gay, is that true?"

To me, that was hurtful and embarrassing. I felt like I wanted to die, but I never let anyone know how I was really feeling. I just made myself go completely numb to the hurt, only feeling anger. But it didn't work because all my other feelings continued to build up, colliding and swarming around like the winds of an unpredictable storm.

I was rude to the other residents for the littlest things. Like when one asked if he could have some of my cereal, I responded, "Why the hell would I give you something of mine?" He just rolled his eyes and walked away. Another resident asked if I had a bar of soap he could borrow. I said, "Do I look like your freakin' mother to you?" He just started mumbling and walked away, too.

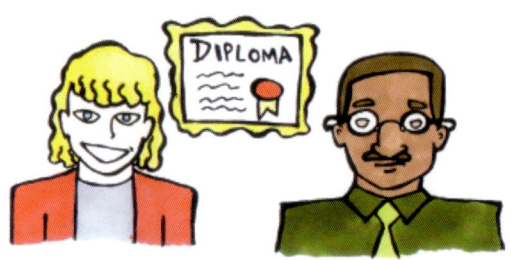

My anger was a reflection of how much I was hurting inside. Because I was hurting so badly and didn't want anyone to know, I became more and more angry, and that's when Dr. K really got down to business. She told me she thought I was trying to get at people's most sensitive, vulnerable sides, so I could make them feel the way I felt. Then she began to dig deeper. Instead of just telling me not to act out anymore, she asked me why I did it. How did it make me feel to insult someone? Did I think it was a positive thing to do?

At first I didn't know what to say to her questions because they were so direct. I explained to her that the things they said about me really hurt. And it wasn't just the fact that they weren't true. It was that some of the same people saying these things claimed to be my friends.

But I also liked that she was willing to be so direct with me. With questions like that, I knew we were getting somewhere and that I was dealing with someone who cared. Which is what I wanted all along—someone who was going to be there whenever I needed her. Someone who understood both sides of the story.

Working with Dr. K, I learned not to get so angry at so many little things. She helped me uncover a side of myself I never knew I had and showed me how to look at myself from the outside in. With her help, I realized that the ways I was acting were just a cover for my true feelings.

I realized that the ways I was acting were just a cover for my true feelings.

I still have to work on expressing my feelings more and not always thinking someone is talking badly about me. I still have to work on watching the things I say or at least how I say them, which may take a while. But Dr. K also helped me see that the things that went on at my group home weren't all my fault, and what was my fault I'd have to admit to. And she helped me realize that I actually did have a reason to live.

Dr. K helped me beyond words. She was the only person I trusted. So it really hurt me the day I found out she was leaving. I just felt like shutting out everything around me.

It's going to be hard to start with another therapist because I don't feel like going back and talking about my past after doing it with four other therapists. I just want to move forward.

I need someone I feel I can trust, with whom I can really talk about myself and my life. Sometimes, I just need to talk about me. Just me.

Norman was 16 when he wrote this story.

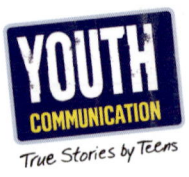

Who We Are
(and why we wrote this booklet)

Youth Communication, founded in 1980, runs an intensive writing and publishing program for teenagers in New York City. Many teenagers who have participated in our program are struggling with mental health issues such as depression, anxiety, ADD, and cutting. Others are dealing with more general life problems. They may feel sad because they had to leave their friends behind when they moved here from another country, or because their parents work such long hours they cannot provide much support.

Some of those teens are in therapy or other kinds of counseling. Some are taking medication. Some have gotten help through hospitalizion. Others are using self-help techniques, like exercise or writing. And many are finding help from informal sources like friends and mentors.

While many of the teens are happy with the help they are getting, others are dissatisfied or confused. Some of them desperately want help but don't know where to find it. Others are getting therapy or medication they may not want or understand.

We wrote this booklet to explain the real deal about getting help. More than a dozen teens worked on it and made countless suggestions to insure that the booklet is clear and is respectful of your experiences.

Many adult professionals also reviewed the booklet to make sure that it is factually correct and that it reflects their experiences too. We hope that it explains mental health services in a way that helps you, the teen reader, get the services you need to get the most out of your life.